ZAKARIA MERAD
SAMIA MERAD
HOURIA BELKRALLADI

Practical manual of endometrial pathology

ZAKARIA MERAD
SAMIA MERAD
HOURIA BELKRALLADI

Practical manual of endometrial pathology

Functional and tumoral pathologies of the endometrium

ScienciaScripts

Imprint

Cover image: www.ingimage.com

This book is a translation from the original published under ISBN 978-620-6-71758-4.

Publisher:
Sciencia Scripts
is a trademark of
Dodo Books Indian Ocean Ltd. and OmniScriptum S.R.L publishing group

120 High Road, East Finchley, London, N2 9ED, United Kingdom
Str. Armeneasca 28/1, office 1, Chisinau MD-2012, Republic of Moldova, Europe
Printed at: see last page
ISBN: 978-620-7-90724-3

PRACTICAL MANUAL ON ENDOMETRIAL PATHOLOGY

ZAKARIA MERAD SAMIA MERAD

HOURIA BELKRALLADI

PREFACE

Anatomy and cytology pathology plays an increasingly important role in modern medicine. In addition to its traditional diagnostic role, it now plays a major role in the therapeutic management of many diseases.

This treatise on endometrial pathology contains everything a senior or resident pathologist needs to know about this pathology. It is also aimed at gynaecologists and oncologists to help them better understand this pathology.

The text is concise, with the explanations necessary for understanding, learning and retaining.

This treatise is essential for doctors if they are to make a successful diagnosis of endometrial pathology.

AMAL HAMHAMI

LIST OF AUTHORS

Zakaria MERAD

Senior Lecturer, Faculty of Medicine, Djilali Liabes University,

Department of Pathological Anatomy and Cytology, Sidi Bel Abbes University Hospital, ALGERIA

Samia MERAD

Assistant Professor, Faculty of Medicine, Djilali Liabes University,

Occupational Medicine Department, Sidi Bel Abbes University Hospital, ALGERIA

Houria BELKRALLADI

Professor, Faculty of Medicine, Djilali Liabes University,

Department of Pathological Anatomy and Cytology, Sidi Bel Abbes University Hospital, ALGERIA

TABLE OF CONTENTS

INTRODUCTION

The study of endometrial pathology aims to provide a general overview of this complex and important subject in gynaecology. It will address the different facets of this pathology, including its definition, its impact on women's health and approaches to management. Functional endometrial pathology refers to a group of disorders that affect the inner layer of the uterus, the endometrium. These disorders include hyperplasia, atrophy, abnormal bleeding and hormonal imbalances. This detailed definition will provide a better understanding of the clinical implications of this condition. Endometrial tumour pathology is essential and of major importance in understanding the characteristics, types and treatments of endometrial tumours. This section will provide an overview of the fundamental aspects of this pathology, including risk factors, clinical presentation, diagnosis, treatment, prognosis and recent research. It is also an opportunity to raise awareness among healthcare professionals of the importance of early detection o f precancerous states of atypical hyperplasia to ensure better management by offering tailored and personalised care.The importance of studying endometrial tumour pathology lies in its contribution to the prevention, early diagnosis and effective treatment of endometrial cancer.

FUNCTIONAL PATHOLOGY OF THE ENDOMETRIUM

The endometrium is a tissue that covers the inner part of the uterus and plays an important role during pregnancy. It undergoes architectural and cytological changes depending on the phase of the menstrual cycle, under the influence of sex hormones (oestrogen and progesterone). Examination of the normal endometrium and its different phases is very important for two reasons; the first is to look for abnormal changes (metaplasia or neoplasia) and the second, especially in women in the reproductive phase, is to determine the date of ovulation and the progression of the luteal phase.

1/ NORMAL ENDOMETRAL ' Histological aspect

1.1. Early proliferation of the uterus after menstruation

- Glands are round to tubular with rare mitoses and subtle nuclear stratification
- The chorion is dense

1.2. Proliferative uterus

- Regularly spaced round to tubular glands with pseudostratified, elongated and hyperchromatic nuclei
- The surrounding chorion is dense and slightly oedematous; the cells are uniform, round or even fusiform.
- The gland/chorion ratio is <1 (glands represent less than 50% of the surface area)
- Mitoses are marked in the epithelium of the glands and the chorion.

1.3. Peri-ovulatory uterus (16ème day)

- The glands are slightly tortuous tubular with pseudostratified nuclei and scattered supra-nuclear (basal) vacuoles (in < 50% of the cells of each gland).
- Mitoses are easily identifiable in the glands and chorion

1.4. Early secretory uterus (vacuolisation of the glands)

- Day 17: diffuse supra-nuclear vacuolisation in > 50% of the cells in each gland (piano key pattern); mitoses are rare or absent
- Day 18: sub- and supra-nuclear vacuoles, the nuclei are generally located in the median part of the cytoplasm
- Day 19: Mostly supra-nuclear vacuoles with the appearance of intra-luminal secretions; the nuclei are in a basal position and there is no mitotic activity.

1.5. Semi-secretory uterus (intra-luminal glandular secretion and oedema of the chorion)

- Day 20: a peak in intra-luminal secretions with increased glandular tortuosity and uniform congestion; occasional supra-nuclear vacuoles
- Day 21: the chorion shows focal oedema; intra-luminal secretions are still significant
- Day 22: the chorion shows diffuse oedema, mainly perivascular, with naked nuclei (not pre-decidualised).

1.6. Late secretory endometrium (pre-decidualisation of chorion)

- Pre-deciduous change: visible basophilic cytoplasm with round nuclei and fine chromatin
- Day 23: Pre-decidual change limited to the chorion around the spiral arterioles
- Day 24: Pre-decisional changes linking vascular elements and glands
- Day 25: Thin, uneven layer of pre-decisive change beneath the surface
- Day 26: Thick continuous layer of pre-deciduous change below the surface; neutrophils are rare
- Day 27: Diffuse pre-deciduous change over the entire surface with numerous neutrophils

1.7. Menstrual uterus

- The chorion is the site of congestive vessels

- Secretory glands exhausted (irregular shape with collapsed lumens, slight stratification)

- A significant neutrophilic inflammatory infiltrate

2/ GESTATIONAL ENDOMETRIUM

Microscopic aspects :

- The endometrial tissue shows diffuse decidualisation of the chorion (decidua) and prominent secretory glands.

- Arias-Stella reactions: hyper-secreting glands with vacuolisation of cells containing hyperchromatic "upholsterer's nail" nuclei and no mitosis

- Design products (in first-quarter samples)

- Presence of immature chorionic villi

- Membranes: amnion and chorion

- Trophoblast of the recent implantation site (intermediate trophoblast cells mixed with fibrinoid material at the interface with the decidua)

Differential diagnosis

- Intrauterine or extrauterine pregnancy

- Exogenous progestogen effect (lapsed)

- Clear cell adenocarcinoma (vs Arias-Stella reaction)

3/ ENDOMETRIUM UNDER HORMONAL IMPREGNATION MEDICAMENTOUS' Histological aspect'

3.1. Oestrogen

- In pre-menopausal women, excess oestrogen will result in an abnormal proliferative endometrium described as 'anovulatory' or 'disordered proliferative', similar to cases of excess endogenous oestrogen.

- In post-menopausal women, low proliferative activity is observed in an apparently inactive endometrium.

- Long-term exposure carries a risk of developing hyperplasia or even neoplasia.

3.2. Progesterones

- During the first few weeks, the glands and chorion undergo secretory differentiation (similar to the secretory phase).
- In the event of prolonged exposure, the glands become small and inactive, while the chorion remains diffusely pseudo-decidualised.
- After months/years of treatment, the endometrium becomes atrophic

3.3. Oral contraceptives

- Combined oral contraceptives: the histological appearance of the endometrium varies according to the number of cycles administered. When first taken, the endometrium presents an "asynchronous" appearance: the glands are tubular, reminiscent of the proliferative phase, but with vacuolisation and absent mitoses. Over time, there will be pseudo-decidualisation and secretory glandular changes. After many intakes, the glands exhaust their secretions and gradually become small and atrophic, while the chorion remains diffuse and pseudo-decidualised.

3.4. Hormone replacement therapy (HRT)

- Cyclic HRT leads to proliferative secretory changes and "delayed" during the oestrogenic and progestagenic phases of the artificial cycle respectively
- Combined HRT leads to atrophy or changes linked to progestin impregnation

3.5. Selective oestrogen receptor modulators

- Tamoxifen induces atrophy or oestrogenic changes due to its weak oestrogen receptor agonist property. Raloxifene induces atrophy

-Ovulation induction therapy (clomiphene): altered secretory differentiation with persistent vacuolisation, less glandular tortuosity and reduced pre-decidualisation.

3.6. Progesterone receptor modulators

- Significant glandular cystic dilatation with a secretory appearance.

3.7. Gonadotropin agonists, aromatase inhibitors, corticosteroids

- Atrophic uterus

4/ ENDOMETRIAL POLYP

Definition

- Benign exophytic neoplastic proliferation of the endometrial chorion with a non-neoplastic glandular component

Incidence and location

- Relatively common
- Risk factors include obesity, hypertension and tamoxifen use.

Breakdown by age

- Peak incidence fifth decade

Clinical characteristics

- Abnormal bleeding,

Radiological characteristics

- Polypoid or sessile mass on ultrasound or hysteroscopy

Prognosis and treatment

- Favourable prognosis after excision

Macroscopy

- An ovoid or elongated stalked or sessile mass with a firm to fleshy consistency
- Solid and/or cystic appearance on section

Microscopy

- Irregular glandular architecture with cysts and variations in size and shape
- Chorionic changes (often with increased fibrosis and collagen deposits)
- Thick-walled vessels

Molecular analysis

- Chorion cells have rearrangements in HMGC-Y (HMGA) and HGMI-C

Differential diagnosis

- Low-grade Müller adenosarcoma
- Atypical polypoid adenomyoma
- Normal uterus

5/ ENDOMETRITIS

Definition

- Non-physiological inflammation of the endometrium post-partum or post-abortion

Incidence

- Pregnancy-related endometritis more common after caesarean section (13% to

90%) than vaginal delivery (1% to 3%).

Breakdown by age

- Childbearing age and peri-menopausal women

Clinical characteristics

- Pregnancy-related endometritis generally occurs shortly after an abortion
- Acute presentation with discharge, bleeding and systemic symptoms (fever)
- Non-obstetric endometritis associated with pelvic inflammatory disease
- Contributing factors include the intrauterine device
- Intermenstrual bleeding and infertility

Prognosis and treatment

- Antibiotic therapy of choice
- Surgery for complicated pelvic inflammatory disease or pyometra

Macroscopy

- Generally undetectable (except pyometra)

Microscopy

- Pregnancy-related: extensive confluent inflammation with necrotic tissue
- Acute endometritis: prominent neutrophilic infiltrates with microabscesses
- Chronic endometritis: plasma cells in the endometrium (generally superficial and focally confluent, around the vessels)
- Generally mixed with lymphocytes, lymphoid aggregates, and eosinophils
- Reactive glandular changes (lack of response to hormones and metaplasia)
- Fibrosis and/or oedema of the chorion

Differential diagnosis

- Normal post-partum/post-abortion uterus

- Menstrual uterus

6/ ANOVULATION

Definition

- Cessation or suppression of ovulation

Incidence

- Most frequent cause of abnormal uterine bleeding in the pre- and peri-menopausal period (77%)

Clinical characteristics

- More frequent during the peri-menopause (physiological deterioration in ovarian function)
- In younger patients, in the context of polycystic ovary syndrome or other endocrine imbalances, including obesity

Radiological characteristics

- Thickened endometrial mucosa

Prognosis and treatment

- Hormone therapy

Macroscopy

- Irregularly thickened endometrial wall

Microscopy

Anovulation associated with persistent unopposed oestrogen production (disordered proliferative endometrium):

- Glands of irregular shape and distribution, with dilated glands
- The chorion is dense with focal fibrin thrombi

Anovulation associated with follicular failure and low oestrogen levels :

- Tubular glands with caryorrhexis

Differential diagnosis

- Endometrial polyp
- Dysfunctional ovulatory cycles (corpus luteum failure)
- Non-atypical endometrial hyperplasia
- Endometrioid intraepithelial neoplasia

7/ ENDOMETRIAL METAPALSIA

Definition

- Endometrial differentiation resembling other epithelial phenotypes in the mucosal tract

Breakdown by age

- More frequent in peri-/post-menopausal women and those undergoing exogenous hormonal impregnation

Clinical characteristics

- Generally asymptomatic
- Symptoms (bleeding) occur if they are associated with a pre-neoplastic syndrome.

Squamous metaplasia

- Scaly morulae isolated or with glandular congestion on biopsy
- Follow-up endometrial sampling in 3 to 6 months Microscopy
- Most frequent non-keratinising squamous differentiation
- Small clusters of cells with uniform round nuclei in the centre and eosinophilic cytoplasm generally located in the lumens of the glands

Differential diagnosis

- High-grade cervical squamous intraepithelial lesion
- Endometrial neoplasia with squamous differentiation
- Atypical polypoid adenomyoma Mucinous metaplasia
- Architecturally simple metaplasia (type A) considered benign: simple follow-up
- Papillary/micropapillary proliferation (type B) may be associated with concomitant neoplasia; sampling and follow-up over 3 to 6 months.
- Complex cribriform, papillary and microglandular architecture (type C) associated with a high risk of malignancy

Microscopy

- Type A: a coating of mucinous epithelium
- Type B: focal papillae and micropapillae
- Type C: papillae and cribriforms Tubal metaplasia and eosinophils
- Low risk of associated carcinoma in the absence of complexity
- Higher risk of carcinoma in cases of complex architecture. Follow-up biopsy within 3 to 6 months

Microscopy

- Glandular epithelium with densely pink granular cytoplasm. Simple cuboid architecture or complex papillary and/or microacinar proliferations.
- In the context of repair, the eosinophilic change involves the endometrial surface

Differential diagnosis

- Endometrial neoplasia with eosinophilic metaplasia Syncytial papillary metaplasia
- Simple morphology considered benign

- Complex architectural morphologies associated with a high risk of malignancy

Microscopy

- Superficial syncytial papillary metaplasia: benign process observed in the context of endometrial degradation (malformed micropapillaries) and on the surface of endometrial polyps.
- Stratified cells with indistinct cell borders, moderate cytoplasm and loss of nuclear polarity, forming a syncytium commonly associated with eosinophilic and mucinous metaplasia.

Intraglandular papillary metaplasia: divided into simple (short, unbranched, with a low risk of malignancy) and complex (diffuse, branched and crowded papillae, with a high risk of endometrioid malignancy)

Differential diagnosis

- Serous endometrial carcinoma

GLANDULAR ENDOMETRIAL TUMOUR PATHOLOGY 1/ NON-ATYPICAL ENDOMETRIAL HYPERPLASIA

Definition:

- Endometrial glandular proliferation characterised by increased glandular density
- Secondary to excessive oestrogen stimulation

Incidence and location :

- Common (150,000 to 200,000 new cases diagnosed each year in Western Europe)

Morbidity and mortality :

- Low risk of progression to carcinoma (2-4%)

- The risk increases if the excess oestrogen persists over time

Breakdown by sex, race and age :

- Generally in peri-menopausal women

- Young women and teenagers are less common

Clinical features :

- Most frequent abnormal vaginal bleeding, sometimes asymptomatic (diagnosed incidentally)

Prognosis and treatment:

- Hormonal therapy (progestins)

Macroscopy :

- Irregular thickening of the endometrium

Microscopy :

- Increase in endometrial glandular volume of more than 50% of the surface (gland to chorion ratio > 1)
- The glands are round and tubular, some with irregular contours (angular, cystic).
- Polarity-preserved nuclear pseudostratification (similar to proliferative phase)
- Chorion loose but present between the glands
- No atypia

Differential diagnosis:

- Variations/artefacts of the endometrium in a normal cycle
- Anovulatory cycles/disordered proliferative endometrium
- Cystic atrophy
- Endometrial polyp
- Metaplasias of the endometrium
- Atypical endometrial hyperplasia
- Well-differentiated endometrioid carcinoma

2/ ATYPICAL ENDOMETRIAL HYPERPLASIA

Definition:

- Endometrial glandular proliferation characterised by an increase in the number of glands

Incidence and location :

- Present in 1.2 to 1.4% of endometrial biopsies

Morbidity and mortality:

- 38% risk of carcinoma
- 45 times greater risk of developing carcinoma over time

Breakdown by sex, race and age :

- Generally peri- and post-menopausal
- Women of childbearing age are less affected

Clinical features :

- Abnormal vaginal bleeding and post-menopausal bleeding are the most common.
- Abnormal uterus on ultrasound (thickened or polypoid)

Prognosis and treatment:

- Hysterectomy with bilateral adnexectomy is the curative treatment if there is no associated malignant tumour.
- High-dose progestins in cases of infertility
- Treatment includes continuous hormone therapy for at least 6 months and follow-up with repeated endometrial sampling.

Macroscopy :

- Can appear polypoid or thickening of the endometrial mucosa

Microscopy :

- Glands congested (exceeding 50% of surface area; gland/chorion ratio >1)
- The glands are round to tubular, or increasingly irregular with ramifications, star-shaped or dilated.
- The chorion, although not very abundant,
- Generally pseudostratification with a rounded nucleus and presence of mitoses

Differential diagnosis:

- Variations/artefacts of the endometrium in a normal cycle
- Non-atypical endometrial hyperplasia

- Endometrial polyp

- Metaplasias of the endometrium

- Endocervical mucosa showing reactive changes (squamous metaplasia, microglandular hyperplasia)

- Well-differentiated endometrioid carcinoma

- Endocervical adenocarcinoma

3/ ENDOMETRIAL CARCINOMA

Definition:

- Malignant epithelial tumour of the endometrium

Incidence and location :

- Most common malignant tumour of the female genital tract (10-20%).

- Endometrioid carcinoma 80

- Serous carcinoma 5 -10

- Carcinosarcoma: <5

- Clear cell carcinoma <5

- Other (undifferentiated, dedifferentiated, neuroendocrine) <1

Morbidity and mortality :

- Low-grade endometrioid carcinoma: 5-year survival rate of 85% to 90%.

- High-grade endometrioid/non-endometrioid carcinomas: 30 to 70%.

Breakdown by sex, race and age :

- The incidence appears to be higher in Caucasians Endometrioid: generally peri-menopausal
Non-endometrioid: generally post-menopausal

Clinical features :

- Abnormal vaginal bleeding

- Constitutional symptoms

- Rarely asymptomatic (early lesions)

Prognosis and treatment:

- Poor prognosis:

1. High-grade histology

2. Histological type (high-grade endometrioid, non-endometrioid)

3. Advanced stage

4. Deep invasion of the myometrium

5. Extensive invasion of the lymphovascular space

6. Serosal and adnexal involvement

7. Lymph node metastases (macrometastases)

8. Molecular group

- A high copy number (abnormal p53) has the worst prognosis

- POLE mutation has an excellent prognosis

Treatment

- Hysterectomy with bilateral adnexectomy is the treatment of choice

- If high risk, +/- pelvic and para-aortic lymphadenectomy, omentectomy, and adjuvant radiotherapy

- If advanced, progestins and/or chemotherapy

Macroscopy :

- Normal or enlarged uterus

- Localised polypoid mass (usually posterior wall)

- Discrete nodules or plaques with variable thickening

- Primary lower uterine segment, particularly in Lynch syndrome

- White scaly appearance if extensive squamous differentiation

- Gelatinous or mucoid appearance if mucinous differentiation

Microscopy :

- Endometrioid adenocarcinoma: variable resemblance to normal endometrial glands depending on the degree of differentiation
- FIGO grade based on glandular and solid (but not scaly) components

Grade 1: <5% solid growth (low grade) Grade 2: 5 to 50% solid growth (low grade) Grade 3: >50% solid growth (high grade)

- Severe nuclear atypia increases the grade Variants of endometrioid adenocarcinoma :
- With squamous differentiation: Morules (without keratin), large irregular nests with intercellular bridges (keratinised), clear cytoplasm
- Papillary (villoglandular, papillary NOS)
- Secretory

Variant : Mucinous adenocarcinoma

- > 50% of cells containing intra-cytoplasmic mucin
- Cytology generally low grade and complex architecture

Immunohistochemistry

- Pancytokeratin, EMA CK7, vimentin generally positive Low-grade endometrioid carcinoma (FIGO grades 1 and 2) :
- ER, PR positive (generally diffuse and strong)
- P 53 normal (wild type)
- p16 negative

High-grade endometrioid carcinoma (FIGO grade 3) :

- Overexpression of p53 and p16 in approximately 30
- Chromogranin A, synaptophysin and CD56 may be focally positive
- 40% loss of BAF250a (ARID1A)

Molecular analysis

- Low-grade endometrioid carcinoma: Mutations in KRAS, ARID1A, PTEN and CTNNB1

Low mutational load and low number of copy number variations Frequent microsatellite instability and MMR deficiency

- High-grade endometrioid carcinoma :

Heterogeneous group: mix of low copy number, high copy number (abnormal p53), hyper-mutated (MMR deficient)

Differential diagnosis:

Low-grade endometrioid carcinoma :

- Atypical polypoid adenomyoma
- Syncytial papillary metaplasia of the endometrium
- Metastatic tumours (colon and breast the most common) Endometrioid carcinoma with mucinous differentiation :
- Endocervical microglandular hyperplasia
- Mucinous metaplasia or endometrium
- Endocervical adenocarcinoma (HPV-related, gastric) High-grade endometrioid carcinoma :
- Serous carcinoma
- Clear cell carcinoma
- Carcinosarcoma
- Undifferentiated/differentiated carcinoma

3.1. SEROUS ENDOMETRIAL CARCINOMA

Macroscopy:

- Normal-sized or markedly enlarged uterus
- May be confined to a polyp or not visible
- Irregular polypoid or papillary mass

Microscopy :

- Papillae of irregular size and shape with prominent cell buds
- Glandular with narrowed and irregular lumina (slit or starfish shaped) due to cell stratification and loss of nuclear polarity
- Solid

Cytological appearance :

- Large, pleomorphic cells
- High nuclear/cytoplasmic ratio
- Coarse chromatin and prominent nucleoli
- Intense mitotic activity and abundant apoptotic bodies
- Psammoma bodies (up to 30%)
- Diagram of gaping glands of myometrial +/- lymphovascular invasion

Immunohistochemistry

- Pancytokeratin, CK7, EMA, PAX8 positive
- BEP4, B72.3, vimentin positive
- Abnormal P53 (overexpression or no phenotype)
- Strong and diffuse p16 expression
- WT1 generally negative
- ER expression, PR generally low
- Napsin-A and AMACR negative

Molecular analysis

- TP53 mutations (early pathogenic event)
- Belongs to the high copy number category (abnormal p53)

Pathological differential diagnosis :

- Low-grade endometrioid carcinoma
- High-grade endometrioid carcinoma
- Clear cell carcinoma
- Carcinosarcoma
- Undifferentiated carcinoma

3.2. ENDOMETRIAL CLEAR CELL CARCINOMA

Macroscopy :

- Diffuse or polypoid
- Friable
- Often haemorrhage and necrosis

Microscopy :

- Papillary (most common): papillae often small, hyalinised or oedematous/myxomatous
- Tubulocystic
- Solid

Cytological characteristics

- Clear/oxyphilic cells
- Flattened and cubic cells also common
- Intra-luminal eosinophilic or basophilic secretions
- Targeted cells (intra-cytoplasmic eosinophilic cells: PAS-positive, resistant to

diastase) hyaline bodies)

- High-grade but relatively uniform nuclei with prominent nucleoli
- Frequent mitosis
- +/- Inflammatory neutrophil/plasmacytic infiltrate

Immunohistochemistry :

- PAX 8, CK7, CAM5.2, 34 β E12 and BerEP4 generally positive
- HNF1β (100%), Napsin-A (90%), AMACR (75%) positive
- (Napsin-A the most specific)
- Loss of BAF250a expression
- overexpression of p16 in approximately 50% of cases
- CK 20, WT1 generally negative
- ER and PR generally negative
- Abnormal MMR in 20% (generally loss of MSH6)

Molecular analysis

- Mutations in ARID1A, PIK3CA, TP53
- Separation according to TCGA molecular classification: 6% POLE mutated, 20% MMR deficient,

Differential diagnosis:

- Arias-Stella reaction
- Reactive changes due to surface repair
- Endometrioid carcinoma
- Serous carcinoma
- Adenomatoid tumour
- Placental trophoblastic tumour
- Epithelioid smooth muscle tumour

- PEComa

- Alveolar soft tissue sarcoma

3.3. INDIFFERENT ENDOMETRIAL CARCINOMA

Macroscopy :

- Soft, crumbly exophytic mass

Microscopy:

- Tumour cells arranged in malformed sheets or trabeculae
- Monotonous population of non-cohesive cells with high-grade characteristics (high N:C ratio, nucleoli, frequent mitoses, necrosis)

Immunohistochemistry :

- Positive EMA, generally focal
- Cytokeratins (in particular CK8/18) generally focal
- E-cadherin generally negative
- PAX 8, ER and PR negative
- Abnormal MMR (MLH1/PMS2 loss) in 50% of cases

Differential diagnosis:

- High-grade endometrioid carcinoma (FIGO grade 3)
- Carcinosarcoma
- Neuroendocrine carcinoma (small cell type)
- Lymphoma
- Serous carcinoma
- Undifferentiated uterine sarcoma
- High-grade endometrial stromal sarcoma

3.4. ENDOMETRIAL CARCINOMA, NEUROENDOCRINE TYPE

Macroscopy :

- Often large and polypoid
- Frequent necrosis and haemorrhage

Microscopy :

Small cell carcinoma :

- Broadcast
- Embedded
- Trabecular
- Not very cohesive
- Round to ovoid cells
- High nuclear/cytoplasmic ratio
- Dark, agglomerated chromatin
- Frequent moulding and apoptotic bodies
- Intense mitotic activity
- Frequent necrosis, frequent myometrial and lymphovascular invasion Large cell neuroendocrine carcinoma :
- Embedded
- Wide, corded trabeculae +/- nuclear palisade
- Large round to polygonal cells
- Vesicular or hyperchromatic nuclei with prominent nucleoli
- Intense mitotic activity
- Common geographic, myometrial and lymphovascular necrosis

Immunohistochemistry :

- Chromogranin A, synaptophysin, CD 56 are positive

- Pancytokeratin, CK18 positive
- PAX8 and p16 may be positive
- TTF1 rarely positive

Differential diagnosis :

- Small cell carcinoma of the uterine cervix
- Undifferentiated/differentiated carcinoma
- Primary neuroectodermal tumour
- Lymphoma

4/ ENDOMETRIAL CARCINOSARCOMA

Definition:

- High-grade malignant tumour composed of malignant epithelial and mesenchymal cells.

Impact :

- 5% of malignant tumours of the uterus

Breakdown by breed and age

- Post-menopausal women (average age 65)
- 5% in patients aged ≤50 years

Clinical characteristics

- Postmenopausal bleeding
- Enlarged uterus and/or pelvic pain
- History of radiotherapy in up to 37% of women

Prognosis and treatment

- 5-year survival rate of 5 to 35% for all stages (median survival 2 years for all stages)

- 5-year survival rate of 40-60% for stage I-II tumours
- The tumour extends outside the uterus (stages III to IV) at the time of diagnosis in two-thirds of cases.
- Higher risk of metastasis if serous or clear cell components
- A heterologous sarcomatous component has a poor prognosis
- Total hysterectomy with bilateral adnexectomy is the mainstay of treatment
- Cisplatin-based chemotherapy and radiotherapy usually recommended

Macroscopy :

- Large polypoid masses occupying the uterine cavity +/- prolapse through the endocervical canal
- The cut looks fleshy
- Frequent haemorrhage and necrosis with formation of secondary cysts

Microscopy :

Mixture of high-grade carcinomatous and sarcomatous components

Carcinomatous component :

- Serous, high-grade endometrioid, clear-cell, most frequent Sarcomatous component :
- Homologous or heterologous
- Endometrial stromal sarcoma, leiomyosarcoma and undifferentiated sarcoma
- uterine sarcoma most frequent homologous types: rhabdomyosarcoma and chondrosarcoma most frequent heterologous types

Immunohistochemistry :

- Cytokeratin, EMA, CK8/18 and E-cadherin strongly positive for the carcinomatous component
- P53 and p16 are focally positive in both components

Differential diagnosis :

- Low-grade fusiform endometrioid carcinoma
- High-grade endometrioid carcinoma
- Undifferentiated and dedifferentiated serous clear cell carcinoma
- Undifferentiated endometrial sarcoma
- Leiomyosarcoma
- Müller adenosarcoma

UTERINE MESENCHYMAL TUMOUR PATHOLOGY

The spectrum of uterine mesenchymal tumours and the mixed mesenchymal-epithelial type has expanded in recent years, largely due to the cumulative experience reported in larger case series, as well as the identification of recurrent problems of gene fusions and other molecular alterations. In current practice, the approach to most mesenchymal neoplasms encountered in the uterus begins with a judicious morphological examination, which in many cases is sufficient for diagnosis.

1/ CONVENTIONAL LEIOMYOMA AND ITS VARIANTS

Definition

- Benign tumour of the smooth muscles of the uterus

Incidence

- Most common tumour in women
- Present in 70% of hysterectomy specimens

Breakdown by breed and age

- Occurs in 40-50% of women over 40 and 20-30% of women under 30.
- Higher incidence in black women

Clinical characteristics

- Symptomatic in a third of patients
- Abnormal uterine bleeding and dysmenorrhoea
- Abdominal pain and/or pressure
- Infertility, frequent spontaneous abortions and pregnancy-related problems.
- Rarely ascites (pseudo-Meigs syndrome)

Prognosis and treatment

- Benin
- Definitive treatment by hysterectomy
- Myomectomy
- Pharmacological treatment includes GnRH agonists and selective progesterone modulators.
- Complications include recurrence after treatment has been stopped, infection and uterine rupture.

Macroscopy :

- Variable size (can be > 25 cm), often multiple
- Location: intramural, submucosal or subserosal
- Submucosal tumours often accompanied by superficial ulceration and haemorrhage
- Sub-serous pedunculated tumours may detach and adhere to other pelvic organs (parasitic leiomyoma).
- Degenerative changes include oedema, pseudocystic disease, calcification and haemorrhage.

Conventional leiomyoma: surface: firm, white/grey Variants of leiomyoma:

- Highly cellular leiomyoma, epithelioid leiomyoma: soft, beige to yellow
- Myxoid leiomyoma: soft gelatinous
- Lipoleiomyoma: heterogeneous appearance with soft yellow areas
- Dissecting leiomyoma: worm-like processes in the myometrium or uterine vessels (intravascular intrusion)
- Cotyledonoid leiomyoma: bulging outline resembling the surface of the placenta
- Diffuse leiomyomatosis: diffuse hypertrophy of the uterine wall containing small, ill-defined nodules ($\leq$ 1 cm)

Microscopy :

- Well circumscribed Conventional leiomyoma :
- Normocellular (nuclear density similar to that of normal myometrium)
- Crossed bundles of spindle cells
- Abundant eosinophilic cytoplasm
- Elongated "cigar"-shaped nuclei (tapered ends) if cut longitudinally, ovoid with perinuclear vacuole if cut transversely
- ± Nuclear fence
- Prominent vascular system with numerous thick-walled blood vessels
- Mild to absent cytological atypia and low mitotic index (<5 mitoses/10HPF)
- Reactive/degenerative changes :

Ischaemic necrosis: devitalised areas with progressive accumulation of collagen with a dense hyalinised appearance, transition to viable areas with an increasing cellularity gradient, tissue granulation, haemorrhage and inflammation.

Edema (hydropic change) with pseudocystic cavitation, haemorrhage, focal myxoid change

- Changes related to pregnancy and treatment :

Pregnancy/progestins: haemorrhage, muscle hypertrophy, hyalinisation, myxoid changes (including vessel walls), mitotic activity and hypercellularity around areas of matrix degeneration.

GnRH agonists, ulipristal: apoptosis, hyalinisation, inflammation, vascular necrosis

Arterial embolisation: ischaemic necrosis, fibrosis, foreign body with giant cell reaction

MRI-guided ablation: well-defined necrosis of tumour cells Variants of leiomyoma

- Cellular leiomyoma: higher cellularity than background myometrium
- Highly cellular leiomyoma: cellularity close to endometrial stroma
- Mitotically active leiomyoma: increased mitotic activity (5 to 15 mitoses/10 HPF)
- Epithelioid leiomyoma: polygonal to round cells with numerous eosinophilic cells; cytoplasm (at least 50% of tumour volume) in sheets, nests, cords and trabeculae; slight cytological atypia, <5 mitoses/10HPF, no tumour necrosis.
- Myxoid leiomyoma: myxoid matrix (at least 50% of tumour volume) non-infiltrative borders, slight cytological atypia, <2 mitoses/10HPF, no tumour necrosis
- Leiomyoma with heterologous elements: adipose tissue (lipoleiomyoma), skeletal muscle, bone or cartilage
- Dissecting leiomyoma and cotyledonoid leiomyoma: permeative growth in surrounding myometrium, adjacent vessels and/or parametrial tissue; large, thick-walled vessels in loose tissue separating nodules from smooth muscle

Histochemical and immunohistochemical characteristics

- Leiomyomas with ischaemic changes show extensive blue staining, over-colouring with trichrome (collagen) and loss of distribution of pericellular reticulin.
- Alcian blue stain (pH 2.5) positive, if myxoid
- AML, desmin and h-caldesmon are positive
- ER and PR positive (100%)
- Keratin and EMA frequently positive (more epithelioid variant)
- CD10 expression is variable
- Low proliferation index

Molecular analysis

- MED12 mutations in 80% of conventional leiomyomas (12% of cellular leiomyomas)

- Karyotypic abnormalities in 40 to 50% of conventional leiomyomas including t(12;14)(q15;q24) (HMGA2 gene)

Differential diagnosis

- Leiomyosarcoma (vs. mitotically active and dissecting leiomyoma)
- Endometrial stromal sarcoma (vs. cell dissection and cotyledonoid leiomyoma)
- Epithelioid leiomyosarcoma (vs. epithelioid leiomyoma)
- Perivascular epithelioid cell tumour (vs. epithelioid leiomyoma)
- Myxoid leiomyosarcoma (vs. myxoid leiomyoma and leiomyoma with hydropic change)

1.1. BIZARRE CELL LEIOMYOMA

Definition

- Benign smooth muscle tumour with nuclear atypia

Incidence

- Rare

Clinical characteristics

- Average age 45
- Abnormal uterine bleeding, pelvic mass

Prognosis and treatment

- Considered benign (rate of ectopic propagation < 2%)
- Management by hysterectomy or myomectomy + monitoring

Macroscopy :

- Similar to conventional leiomyoma

- May have a soft, yellow appearance, haemorrhage and cavitation

Microscopy :

- Atypical/bizarre cells: nuclear hypertrophy, irregular nuclear contour, multinucleation, hyperchromasia or coarse chromatin, prominent nucleoli
- Distribution of bizarre cells: diffuse (30%), multifocal (44%), focal (26%)
- Round eosinophilic cytoplasmic inclusions
- Nuclei with a prominent eosinophilic nucleolus surrounded by a perinucleolar halo
- Alveolar oedema

Immunohistochemical characteristics

- Expression of smooth muscle markers and hormone receptors

Molecular analysis

- Molecular profile is similar to that of leiomyosarcomas

Differential diagnosis

- Uterine leiomyosarcoma
- Uterine leiomyoma

2/ UTERINE LEIOMYOSARCOMA

Definition:

- Malignant smooth muscle tumour of the uterus

Incidence

- 1 to 2% of all malignant tumours of the uterus

- Most common sarcoma of the gynaecological tract (> 50% of all sarcomas)

Breakdown by breed and age

- Average age 60 (peri-menopausal and post-menopausal)
- More common in black women

Clinical characteristics

- Abnormal vaginal bleeding
- Abdominal distension, pelvic pain or pressure
- Sometimes hypercalcaemia and eosinophilia
- Rarely, a history of radiotherapy or tamoxifen treatment

Prognosis and treatment

- 5-year survival rate of 15 to 65% depending on stage (best in stage I disease)
- Other prognostic factors: age, tumour size, vascular invasion
- Recurrence rate of around 70% for stages I and II and almost 100% for stages III and IV (within 18 months)
- Haematogenous spread to the lungs and liver and lymphatic spread
- Myxoid leiomyosarcoma appears to have worse survival than conventional surgery
- Epithelioid leiomyosarcoma may recur late (> 10 years)
- Treatment included hysterectomy with bilateral adnexectomy,
- Hormonal therapy in the event of disease progression

Macroscopy :

- Large mass (average 10 cm), poorly circumscribed
- On section, fleshy heterogeneous appearance with necrosis and haemorrhage

Microscopy :

- High grade by definition Conventional leiomyosarcoma :
- Irregular, infiltrating growth
- Hypercellularity composed of intersecting fascicles
- Elongated cores with tapered ends ("cigar" shape)
- Morphological criteria for malignancy (at least two) :
- Significant cytological atypia: moderate or severe, multifocal to diffuse enlarged hyperchromatic nuclei with coarse chromatin and irregular nuclear membranes
- Tumour necrosis: on the map
- Mitotic activity ≥10 mitoses/10 HPF: count at least 50 HPF,
- Vascular invasion in 20% of cases

Epithelioid leiomyosarcoma

- ≥50% epithelioid cells (polygonal eosinophilic cytoplasm, central ovoid nucleus)
- Nests, cords or trabeculae; rarely pseudoglandular spaces
- Frequent central hyalinisation
- Significant cytological atypia (as defined for conventional tumours) may be present.
- Morphological criteria of malignancy (one of the following) : Tumour necrosis Mitotic index ≥5 mitoses/10 HPF Myxoid leiomyosarcoma
- The myxoid matrix separates the fascicles and tumour cells,
- Mitotic activity and nuclear atypia may be subtle or absent
- Hyperchromatic fusiform nuclei
- Morphological criteria for malignancy (at least two) :

Invasive tumour border, cell necrosis, cytological atypia or ≥2 mitoses/10 HPF

Histochemical and immunohistochemical characteristics

- Tumour necrosis may be absent
- Alcian Blue pH 2.5 enhances the myxoid matrix
- AML, desmin, caldesmon, are positive (strong and diffuse in conventional variants, less so in epithelioid and myxoid variants)
- Estrogen, progesterone and androgen receptors often positive
- CD10 and C-KIT may be positive
- Keratin and EMA variably positive (more frequent in epithelioid variant)
- High Ki67 (>10%)

Molecular analysis

- Complex and frequent karyotypic chromosomal aberrations
- TP53 and VIPR2 frequently mutated (also RB1, PTEN)
- Absence of C-KIT mutations and ALK rearrangements

Differential diagnosis

- Variants of leiomyoma
- Pleomorphic rhabdomyosarcoma
- Low-grade endometrial stromal sarcoma
- High-grade endometrial stromal sarcoma
- Undifferentiated endometrial sarcoma
- Carcinosarcoma
- Gastrointestinal stromal tumour
- Endometrial carcinoma (endometrioid, serous)
- Perivascular epithelioid cell tumour
- Placental trophoblastic tumour
- Epithelioid trophoblastic tumour
- Inflammatory myofibroblastic tumour

3/ MALIGNANT TUMOUR OF UNCERTAIN MALIGNANT POTENTIAL (STUMP)

Definition

- Uterine smooth muscle tumours that cannot be classified with certainty as benign or malignant

Incidence

- Rare

Breakdown by breed and age

- Average age 45-50

Clinical characteristics

- Similar to leiomyoma
- Sometimes rapid growth

Prognosis and treatment

- Overall recurrence rate 7 to 36
- Hysterectomy is the treatment of choice, followed by long-term monitoring.
- Patients not undergoing hysterectomy should be closely monitored.

Macroscopy :

- Similar to leiomyoma

Microscopy :

- Significant cytological atypia (multifocal or diffuse) and 8-9 mitoses/10 HPF
- Tumours in which tumour necrosis is suspected but not confirmed
- Mitotic activity >15 mitoses/10 HPF
- Epithelioid tumour with significant atypia; equivocal epithelioid features
- Myxoid tumours presenting a single characteristic among the following: atypia,

≥2 mitoses/10 HPF, or necrosis

Molecular analysis

- MED12 mutations are uncommon (11%).

Differential diagnosis

- Leiomyoma
- Leiomyosarcoma
- Perivascular epithelioid cell tumour
- Inflammatory myofibroblastic tumour

4/ ENDOMETRIAL STROMAL NODULE

Definition

- Tumour whose morphology resembles that of the endometrium in the proliferative phase, with no or minimal infiltration and no lymphovascular invasion.

Incidence

- Uncommon

Breakdown by age

- Fifth to sixth decades (median age 47)

Clinical characteristics

- Abnormal post-menopausal uterine bleeding
- Pelvic or abdominal pain

Prognosis and treatment

- Excellent prognosis
- Subtotal hysterectomy is necessary for diagnosis and is also a definitive

treatment.

Macroscopy :

- A well-defined solitary mass
- Variable size, generally less than 10 cm
- When cut: yellowish appearance, not domed

Microscopy :

- Well-defined, non-encapsulated, highly cellular lesion
- Smooth, generally non-infiltrative interface with the adjacent myometrium
- Border irregularity each measuring less than 3 mm (measured from the entire outer contour of the tumour) with no obvious invasion or vascular invasion
- Uniform population of cells with little cytoplasm
- Spindle to ovoid nuclei with uniform chromatin and inconspicuous nucleoli
- Nuclear size with minimal variation (two to four times the size of lymphocytes)
- Mitotic index <10/10 HPF
- Vascular system made up of small vessels of uniform size
- Thick-walled blood vessels
- No lymphovascular invasion

Immunohistochemical characteristics

- CD10, WT1, ER and PR positive
- AML, desmin, calponin and caldesmon frequently positive in areas of smooth muscle differentiation

Molecular analysis

- Most common JAZF1-SUZ12 fusion (50% to 65%)

Differential diagnosis

- Cellular leiomyoma

- Uterine tumour resembling a stromal tumour of the sex cords of the ovary
- Low-grade endometrial stromal sarcoma
- High-grade endometrial stromal sarcoma

5/ LOW-GRADE STROMAL SARCOMA

Definition

- Tumour whose morphology resembles that of the endometrium in the proliferative phase and permeative infiltration of the uterine wall and lymphovascular invasion.

Incidence

- 10 to 15% of uterine sarcomas

Breakdown by age

- 52 years (range 40 to 55)

Clinical characteristics

- Abnormal uterine bleeding or pelvic pain
- Uterine hypertrophy

Prognosis and treatment

- 5-year survival rate of around 60-80% (depending on stage >90% in stage I)
- Slowly progressing multiple recurrences, whatever the stage, occurring late in life
- Frequent sites of recurrence: pelvis, abdomen, vagina, lung
- Primary surgical treatment: hysterectomy with bilateral adnexectomy
- Hormonal treatment if recurrent or advanced stage

Macroscopy :

- Uterine mass with irregular margins and enlargement of the uterine wall

- Variable tumour size (from <5 to >15 cm)

- On cutting: yellowish in appearance, fleshy

Microscopy :

- Permeative infiltration of the finger-shaped myometrium by expansive nodules
- Frequent invasion of the lymphovascular space
- Morphology of tumour cells and vascular system identical to endometrial stromal nodule
- Histiocytes and hyalinisation may be present
- Necrosis is rare Morphological variations:
- Fibromyxoid: abundant myxoid to fibromatous matrix
- Smooth muscle differentiation: fascicles, some with central collagen (star pattern)
- Stromal differentiation of the sex cords: cords, trabeculae, tubules, retiforms
- Glandular differentiation: structures resembling endometrioid glands
- Rarely: rhabdoid morphology, bizarre cells, giants resembling osteoclasts.

Immunohistochemical characteristics

- ER and PR are strongly and diffusely positive
- CD10 is positive
- AML, desmin and calponin are weakly positive and focal (strong in areas of smooth muscle differentiation)
- SF1, calretinin and inhibin may be positive (stromal differentiation of the sex cords)
- H-Caldesmon, Cyclin D1 and BCOR generally negative
- Proliferation index Ki67 ≤5

Molecular analysis

- Recurrent genetic rearrangements in approximately 55% of cases
- JAZF1-SUZ12 most common in low-grade stromal sarcoma (33-50% of cases)

Differential diagnosis

- Endometrial polyp
- Adenomyosis
- Leiomyosarcoma
- Intravenous leiomyomatosis
- Leiomyoma with intravascular intrusion
- Low-grade mullerian adenosarcoma
- Uterine tumour resembling a tumour of the sex cords of the ovary
- High-grade endometrial stromal sarcoma
- Solitary fibrous tumour
- Gastrointestinal stromal tumour

6/ HIGH-GRADE STROMAL SARCOMA

Definition

- Uterine sarcoma with a more aggressive clinical course than low-grade stromal sarcoma with molecular alterations:
- YWHAE-NUTM2 HG-ESS: YWHAE-NUTM2A/B rearrangements
- BCOR-modified HG-ESS: ZC3H7B-BCOR rearrangement or BCOR ITD

Incidence

- Extremely rare

Breakdown by age

- Wide range, generally peri-menopausal and post-menopausal (average age 50 to 54)

Clinical characteristics

- Abnormal uterine bleeding, pelvic mass
- Ectopic dissemination (advanced stage) frequent (60 to 80% of cases)

Prognosis and treatment

- HG-ESS altered by YWHAE-NUTM2 and BCOR are aggressive tumours
- High risk of rapid recurrence and tumour progression
- Mainly surgical treatment hysterectomy with bilateral adnexectomy
- Chemotherapy and radiotherapy appear to be effective in YWHAENUTM2 HG-ESS mutations

Macroscopy :

- Irregular, soft, fleshy mass, usually with an endometrial base and extension of the submucosal myometrium
- Tumour size: 3-9 cm (median 7.5 cm),
- Necrosis and haemorrhage are frequent

Microscopy :

- Permeative and destructive finger-shaped myometrial invasion

YWHAE-NUTM2 HG-ESS :

- Round cell" component (either exclusive or mixed with a conventional low-grade sarcoma or fibromyxoid component)
- The round cells are epithelioid, with eosinophilic cytoplasm and large nuclei (four to six times the size of the lymphocyte nucleus); prominent nucleoli.
- Tumour necrosis and high mitotic activity (> 10 mitoses/10 HPF)

HG-ESS modified to BCOR :

- Prominent myxoid matrix, sometimes collagenous plaques
- Spindle-shaped cells with elongated hyperchromatic nuclei and mild to moderate atypia
- Marked mitotic activity (> 10 mitoses/10 HPF)

Immunohistochemical characteristics

YWHAE-NUTM2 HG-ESS :

- Component made up of high-grade round cells: BCOR, Cyclin D1 diffusely positive
- CD10, ER, PR are negative
- Low-grade spindle cell component: CD10, ER, PR are positive
- BCOR and Cyclin D1 variably positive
- Weak to negative expression of smooth muscle markers
- Ki67 proliferation index >5% HG-ESS modified in BCOR :
- CD10 positive (strong in ZC3H7B-BCOR HG-ESS fusion, weak in BCOR ITD HG-ESS)
- BCOR and cyclin D1 are positive
- Weak to negative expression of smooth muscle markers
- Variable expression ER and PR

Molecular analysis

- YWHAE-NUTM2 HG-ESS: YWHAE-NUTM2A/B rearrangements
- BCOR-modified HG-ESS: ZC3H7B-BCOR rearrangement or BCOR ITD

Differential diagnosis

YWHAE-NUTM2 HG-ESS :

- Low-grade stromal sarcoma
- Undifferentiated uterine sarcoma

- Undifferentiated endometrial carcinoma

- Epithelioid leiomyosarcoma

HG-ESS modified to BCOR :

- Low-grade stromal sarcoma, fibromyxoid type

- Myxoid leiomyosarcoma

- Undifferentiated uterine sarcoma

7/ INDIFFERENT STROMAL SARCOMA

Definition

- High-grade sarcoma with absence of specific differentiation of the mesenchymal lineage

Incidence

- Rare

Breakdown by age

- Post-menopausal women (average age 60)

Clinical characteristics

- Post-menopausal bleeding

- Fast-growing mass

Prognosis and treatment

- Poor prognosis
- A high number of mitoses (> 25 mitoses/HPF) correlates with poorer survival.
- Frequent ectopic diffusion
- Poor response to systemic treatment

Macroscopy :

- Large fleshy mass (> 10 cm) with heterogeneous appearance when cut

Microscopy :

- Hypercellular tumour with infiltrating margins
- Diffuse leaf-shaped growth with no specific characteristics
- High N:C ratio
- The tumour may be pleomorphic or uniform
- Lack of epithelial or mesenchymal differentiation

Histochemical and immunohistochemical characteristics

- Pericellular reticulin network
- PAX8, epithelial (pan keratin, EMA), smooth muscle (desmin, h-caldesmon, AML) and skeletal muscle (myoglobin, myogenin) markers are negative.
- CD10, ER and PR can be positive

Molecular analysis

- Complex karyotype
- Frequent TP53 mutations
- SMARCA4 mutations in a subset (uniform morphology)

Differential diagnosis

- Undifferentiated and dedifferentiated carcinoma
- Leiomyosarcoma
- HG-ESS (YWHAE-NUTM2)
- Rhabdomyosarcoma
- High-grade adenosarcoma

8/ PRE-VASCULAR EPITHELIOID TUMOUR (PECOM)

Definition

- Tumour composed of cells with a "perivascular epithelioid cell morphology" which co-express smooth muscle and melanocytic markers.

Incidence

- Rare

Breakdown by age

- Women of childbearing age and menopausal women

Clinical characteristics

- Abnormal uterine bleeding

Prognosis and treatment

- Benign, uncertain or malignant behaviour depending on the presence or absence of various pathological variables
- Malignant tumours tend to recur soon after diagnosis
- Total hysterectomy as curative treatment
- Adjuvant therapy and mTOR inhibitors considered in high-risk cases and recurrent tumour

Macroscopy :

- Variable tumour size (1 to >30 cm)
- Well-defined or infiltrating border
- Haemorrhagic appearance on section, rarely necrosis

Microscopy :

- Nests of epithelioid cells and/or fascicles of spindle cells

- Little collagen stroma
- Capillary and small-calibre vessels with perivascular features condensation of tumour cells
- Epithelioid morphology: polygonal cells with eosinophilic granular cytoplasm and round nuclei
- Fascicular growth (similar to smooth muscle) may be observed
- Morphological variants: sclerosing,

Immunohistochemical characteristics

- HMB-45, Melan-A and MITF are positively variable
- Cathepsin-K is positive (100%)
- AML, desmin and h-caldesmon variably positive
- Cytokeratin, inhibin and S-100 are negative

Molecular analysis

- Inactivation of TSC2 and TSC1 (including TSC patients)
- Molecular variants: PECom with TFE3 and RAD51B rearrangements

Differential diagnosis

- Epithelioid smooth muscle tumours
- High-grade stromal sarcoma
- Alveolar soft tissue sarcoma
- Endometrial carcinoma
- Metastatic or primary melanoma

9/ UTERINE RHABDOMYOSARCOMA

Definition

- Malignant mesenchymal tumour of skeletal muscle phenotype

- Three types: embryonic, alveolar, pleomorphic
- Botryoid sarcoma: embryonal rhabdomyosarcoma involving the uterine mucosa (most often the cervix)

Incidence

- Rare in the uterus

Breakdown by age

- Embryonal rhabdomyosarcoma: children and adolescents (botryoid sarcoma), rarely adults
- Pleomorphic and alveolar rhabdomyosarcoma: post-menopausal

Clinical characteristics

- Abnormal bleeding
- Mass extending beyond the cervical os

Prognosis and treatment

- Surgery (complete conservative excision in children, hysterectomy in adults) and adjuvant treatment
- Embryonal rhabdomyosarcoma: good prognosis
- Pleomorphic and alveolar rhabdomyosarcoma: poor prognosis

Macroscopy :

- Botryoid sarcoma: exophytic, lobulated, grape-like appearance

Microscopy :

Embryonal rhabdomyosarcoma :

- Polypoid projections, if botryoid type
- Hypercellular and hypocellular zones, the latter showing myxoid changes
- Submucosal condensation of small round primitive elements of blue cells

("cambial layer"), some with eosinophilic cytoplasmic projections that may show crossed striations ("strap cells").

Alveolar rhabdomyosarcoma :

- Small round blue cells arranged around empty saccular spaces (alveoli)

Pleomorphic rhabdomyosarcoma :

- Numerous rhabdomyoblasts
- Important pleomorphism

Immunohistochemical characteristics

- Desmin, myogenin, MyoD1 are positive
- Hormone receptors are negative

Molecular analysis

- Embryonal rhabdomyosarcoma: DICER1 mutations
- Alveolar rhabdomyosarcoma: PAX3-FKHR or PAX7-FKHR fusion gene

Differential diagnosis

- Carcinosarcoma
- High-grade adenosarcoma
- Leiomyosarcoma
- Fibroepithelial stromal polyp

10/ UTERINE ADENOSARCOMA

Definition

- Mixed mullerian tumour with malignant mesenchymal and benign epithelial components

Incidence

- 5 to 10% of all uterine sarcomas

Breakdown by age

More common in post-menopausal women (median age 58), but can be seen at any age

- 30% of premenopausal women

Clinical characteristics

- Abnormal vaginal bleeding and/or pelvic pain
- Enlarged uterus
- ± History of recurrent endometrial or endocervical polyps

Prognosis and treatment

- Total hysterectomy with bilateral adnexectomy
- 80-90% overall survival rate

Macroscopy :

- Location: endometrium (most common), cervix (9%) or myometrium (4%)
- Average size 5 cm; high-grade lesions generally > 10 cm
- Exophytic soft mass
- Solid appearance when cut (cauliflower-like) ± small cysts

Microscopy :

Biphasic population with the following characteristics throughout the tumour:

- Periglandular stromal condensation ("cuffing")
- Leaf-shaped architecture
- Rigid cystic dilatation
- Cytological stromal atypia (low or high grade)

- ≥2 mitoses/10 HPF Benign glandular component:

- Endometrioid or endocervical epithelium

- ± Epithelial metaplasia Malignant mesenchymal component :

- Low grade: relatively monotonous stromal population (similar to a low-grade stromal sarcoma)

- ± Differentiation of the sex cord or smooth muscles

- High grade: significant pleomorphism (observed at low power), variation greater than twice the size of the endothelial core,

- ± Heterologous elements (most common rhabdomyosarcoma)

- Sarcomatous overgrowth: pure sarcoma representing ≥25% of the tumour

Often superficial myometrial invasion

Immunohistochemical characteristics

- CD10, ER and PR positive (sarcomatous component)

- WT1 is positive (stronger in the case of sarcomatous proliferation)

Molecular analysis

- TP53 mutations in high-grade tumours

- Sarcomatous proliferation associated with global chromosomal instability, high copy number variation, MYBL1 amplification, and ATRX mutations

Differential diagnosis

- Endometrial/endocervical polyp

- Atypical polypoid adenomyoma

- Carcinosarcoma

- Low-grade stromal sarcoma

- High-grade stromal sarcoma

- Undifferentiated uterine sarcoma

- Rhabdomyosarcoma

BIBLIOGRAPHY

Parra-Herran, C., Cesari, M., Djordjevic, B., et al. (2018). Canadian Association of Pathologists-l'Association Canadienne des Pathologists (CAP-ACP) guidelines for benign endometrial biopsy interpretation and reporting. Canadian Journal of Pathology, 10(1), 13-24.

Sakhdari, A., Moghaddam, P. A., & Liu, Y. (2016). Endometrial samples from postmenopausal women: aproposal for adequacy criteria. International Journal of Gynecological Pathology, 35, 525-530.

Sereepapong, W., Suwajanakorn, S., Triratanachat, S., et al (2000) Effects of clomiphene citrate on the endometrium of regularly cycling women. Fertility and Sterility, 73(2), 287-291.

Usluogullari, B., Duvan, C. Z., Usluogullari, C. A. (2015). Use of aromatase inhibitors in practice of gynecology. Journal of Ovarian Research, 8, 4.

Williams, A. R. W., Bergeron, C., Barlow, D. H., Ferenczy, A.(2012). Endometrial morphology after treatment of uterine fibroids with the selective progesterone receptor modulator, ulipristalacetate. International Journal of Gynecological Pathology, 31, 556-569.

Tallini, G., Vanni, R., Manfioletti, G., et al (2000). HMGI-C and HMGI(Y) immunoreactivity correlates with cytogenetic abnormalities in lipomas, pulmonary chondroid hamartomas, endometrial polyps, and uterine leiomyomas and is compatible with rearrangement of the HMGI-C and HMGI(Y) genes. Laboratory Investigation, 80(3), 359-369.

Chen, Y. Q., Fang, R. L., Luo, Y. N., et al. (2016). Analysis of the diagnostic value of CD138 for chronic endometritis, the risk factors for the pathogenesis of chronic endometritis and the effect of chronic endometritis on pregnancy: a cohort study.

BMC Women's Health, 16, 60.

ESHRE Capri Workshop Group (2007). Endometrial bleeding. Human Reproduction Update, 13(5), 421-431.

Ip, P. C., Irving, J. A., Mc Cluggage, W. G., Clement, P. B., Young, R.H. (2013). Papillary proliferation of the endometrium: a clinicopathologic study of 59 cases of simple and complex papillae without cytologic atypia. The American Journal of SurgicalPathology,37, 167-177.

Lehman, M. B., & Hart, W. R. (2001). Simple and complex hyperplastic papillary proliferations of the endometrium: a clinicopathologic study of nine cases of Apparently localized papillary lesions with fibrovascular stromal cores and epithelial metaplasia. The American Journal of Surgical Pathology, 25(11), 1347-1354.

Qiu, W., &Mittal, K. (2003). Comparison of morphologic and immunohistochemical features of cervical microglandular hyperplasia with low grade mucinous adenocarcinoma of the endometrium. International Journal of Gynecological Pathology, 22, 261-265.

Wilson, P. C., Buza, N., & Hui, P. (2016). Progression of endometrial hyperplasia: a revisit under the 2014 WHO classification. International Journal of Clinical and Experimenta lPathology, 9, 1617-1625.

Committee on Gynecologic Practice, Society of Gynecologic Oncology and American College of Obstetricians and Gynecologists (2015) Committee Opinion: Endometrial Intraepithelial Neoplasia. Obstet Gynecol. 125(5):1272-1278.

Baak, J. P., Mutter, G. L., Robboy, S., et al. 2005. The molecular genetics and morphometry-basedendometrialintraepithelialneoplasiaclassification system predicts disease progression in endometrial hyperplasia more accurately than the 1994 World Health Organization classification system. Cancer, 103, 2304-2312.

Yeramian, A., Moreno, G., Dolcet, X., et al. (2013) Endometrial carcinoma: molecular alterations involved in tumor development and progression. Oncogene, 32, 403-413.

Gunderson, C. C. 1, Fader, A. N., Carson, K. A., et al. (2012). Oncologic and reproductive outcomes with progestin therapy in women with endometrial hyperplasia and grade 1 adenocarcinoma: asystematic review. Gynecologic Oncology, 125(2), 477-482.

Hirschowitz, L., Nucci, M., &Zaino, R. J. (2013). Problematic issues in the staging of endometrial, cervical and vulval carcinomas. Histopathology,62(1), 176-202.

Kurnit, K. C., Kim, G. N., Fellman, B. M., et al. (2017). CTNNB1(beta-catenin) mutation identifies low grade, early stage endometrial cancer patients at increased risk of recurrence. Modern Pathology, 30(7), 1032-1041.

Soslow, R. A. (2013). High-grade endometrial carcinomas-strategies for typing. Histopathology, 62, 89-110.

Gatius, S., & Matias-Guiu, X. (2016). Practical issues in the diagnosis of serous carcinoma of the endometrium. Modern Pathology,29(1), S45-S58.

Trinh, V. Q., Pelletier, M. P., Echelard, P., et al. (2019). Distinct Histologic, Immunohistochemical and Clinical Features Associated With Serous Endometrial

Intraepithelial Carcinoma Involving Polyps. Int J Gynecol Pathol. 2019, Advanced Online Publication(PMID 30789501).

DeLair, D. F., Burke, K. A., Selenica, P., et al. (2017). The genetic and scape of endometrial clear cell carcinomas. The Journal of Pathology, 243, 230-241.

Fadare, O., Desouki, M. M., Gwin, K., et al. (2014). Frequent expression of napsin A in clear cell carcinoma of the endometrium: potential diagnostic utility. The American Journal of Surgical Pathology, 38(2), 189-196

Ramalingam, P., Masand, R. P., Euscher, E. D., Malpica, A. (2016).Undifferentiated carcinoma of the endometrium: an expanded immunohistochemical analysis including PAX-8 and basal-like carcinoma surrogate markers. International Journal of Gynecological Pathology, 35(5), 410-418.

Shah, V. I., &Mc Cluggage, W. G. (2015). Cyclin D1 does not distinguishYWHAE- NUTM2 high-grade endometrial stromal sarcoma from undifferentiated endometrial carcinoma. The American Journal of Surgical Pathology, 39(5), 722-724.

Albores-Saavedra, J., Martinez-Benitez, B., Luevano, E. (2008) Small cell carcinomas and large cell neuroendocrine carcinomas of the endometrium and cervix: polypoid tumors and those arising in polyps may have a favorable prognosis.
International Journal of Gynecological Pathology, 27(3), 333-339.

Pocrnich, C. E., Ramalingam, P., Euscher, E. D., Malpica, A.(2016). Neuroendocrine carcinoma of the endometrium: a clinicopathologic study of 25 cases. The American Journal of Surgica lPathology, 40(5), 577-586.

Chiyoda, T., Tsuda, H., Tanaka, H., et al. (2012). Expression profiles of carcinosarcoma of the uterine corpus-are these similar to carcinoma or sarcoma? Genes Chromosomes Cancer, 51(3), 229-329.

Jong, R. A., Nijman, H. W., Wijbrandi, T. F., et al. (2011). Molecular markers and clinical behavior of uterine carcinosarcomas: focus on the epithelial tumor component. Modern Pathology,24(10), 1368-1379.

Ferguson, S. E., Tornos, C., Hummer, A., Barakat, R. R.,Soslow, R.A. (2007). Prognostic features of surgical stage I uterine carcinosarcoma. The American Journal of Surgical Pathology, 31, 1653-1661

Demura, T. A., Revazova, Z. V., Kogan, E. A., et al. (2017). The molecular mechanisms and morphological manifestations of leiomyoma reduction induced by selective progesterone receptor modulators. Arkhiv Patologii, 79(3), 19-26.

Oliva, E. (2016). Practical issues in uterine pathology from banal to bewildering: the remarkable spectrum of smooth muscle neoplasia. Modern Pathology, 29(Suppl. 1), 104-120

Shin, S. J., Kim, J., Lee, S., et al. (2018). Ulipristal acetate induces cell cycle delay and remodeling of extracellular matrix. International Journal of Molecular Medicine, 42(4), 1857-1864

Vilos, G. A., Allaire, C., Laberge, P. Y., et al. (2015). The management of uterine leiomyomas. Journal of Obstetrics and Gynaecology Canada, 37(2), 157-178.

Bennett, J. A., Weigelt, B., Chiang, S., et al. (2017). Leiomyoma with bizarre nuclei: a morphological, immunohistochemical and molecular analysis of 31 cases. Modern Pathology, 30(10), 1476-1488.

Croce, S., Young, R. H., & Oliva, E. (2014). Uterine leiomyomas with bizarre nuclei: a clinicopathologic study of 59 cases. The American Journal of Surgical Pathology, 38, 1330-1339.

Joseph, N. M., Solomon, D. A., Frizzell, N., Rabban, J. T., Zaloudek, C., Garg, K., (2015). Morphology and Immunohistochemistry for 2SC and FH aid in detection of fumarate hydratase gene aberrations in uterine leiomyomas from young patients. The American Journal of Surgical Pathology, 39(11), 1529-1539.

An, Y., Wang, S., & Li, S. (2017). Distinct molecular subtypes of uterine leiomyosarcoma respond differently to chemotherapy treatment. BMC Cancer, 17, 639.

Cuppens, T., Moisse, M., Depreeuw, J. (2018). Integrated genome analysis of uterine leiomyosarcoma to identify novel driver genes and targetable pathways.

International Journal of Cancer, 142(6), 1230-1243.

Ducie, J. A., & Leitao, M. M., Jr. (2016). The role of adjuvant therapy in uterine leiomyosarcoma. Expert Review of Anticancer Therapy, 16(1), 45-55.

Croce, S., Ducoulombier, A., Ribeiro, A., et al. (2018). Genome profiling is an efficient tool to avoid the STUMP classification of uterine smooth muscle lesions: a comprehensive array-genomic hybridization analysis of 77 tumors. Modern Pathology, 31(5), 816-828.

Gupta, M., Laury, A. L., Nucci, M. R., Quade, B. J. (2018). Predictors of adverse outcome in uterine smooth muscle tumours of uncertain malignant potential (STUMP): a clinicopathological analysis of 22 cases with a proposal for the inclusion of additional histological parameters. Histopathology, 73, 284-298.

Chiang, S., et al. (2017). BCOR is a robust diagnostic immunohistochemical marker of genetically diverse high-grade endometrial stromal sarcoma, including tumors exhibiting variant morphology. Modern Pathology, 30(9), 1251-1261.

Chu, P. G., Arber, D. A., Weiss, L. M., et al (2001). Utility of CD10 in distinguishing between endometrial stromal sarcoma and uterine smooth-muscle tumors: an immunohistochemical comparison of 34 cases. Modern Pathology, 14, 465-471.

Hoang, L. N., et al. (2017). Novel high-grade endometrial stromal sarcoma: a morphologic mimicker of myxoid leiomyosarcoma. The American Journal of Surgical Pathology, 41(1), 12-24.

Lee, C. H., Nucci, M. R. (2015). Endometrial stromal sarcoma the new genetic paradigm. Histopathology, 67(1), 1-19.

Seagle, B. L., et al. (2017). Low-grade and high-grade endometrial stromal sarcoma: a National Cancer Database study. Gynecologic Oncology, 146(2),

254-262.

Hardell, E., Josefson, S., Ghaderi, M., et al. (2017). Validation of a mitotic index cutoff as a prognostic marker in undifferentiated uterine sarcomas. The American Journal of Surgical Pathology, 41, 1231-1237.

Hoang, L. N., Lee, Y.-S., Karnezis, A. N., et al. (2016). Immunophenotypic features of dedifferentiated endometrial carcinoma- insights from BRG1/INI1-deficient tumours. Histopathology, 69(4), 560-569.

Kolin, D. L., Dong, F., Baltay, M., et al. (2018). SMARCA4-deficient undifferentiated uterine sarcoma (malignant rhabdoid tumor of the uterus): a clinicopathologic entity distinct from undifferentiated carcinoma. Modern Pathology, 31(9), 1442-1456.

Agaram, N. P., Sung, Y.-S., Zhang, L., et al. (2015). Dichotomy of genetic abnormalities in PEComas with therapeutic implications. The American Journal of Surgical Pathology, 39(6), 813-825.

Bennett, J. A., Braga, A. C., Pinto, A., et al. (2018). Uterine PEComas: a morphologic, immunohistochemical, and molecular analysis of 32 tumors. The American Journal of Surgical Pathology, 42, 1370-1383.

Conlon, N., Soslow, R. A., Murali, R. (2015). Perivascular epithelioid tumours (PEComas) of the gynaecological tract. Journal of Clinical Pathology, 68(6), 418- 426.

Fadare, O. (2008). Perivascular epithelioid cell tumor (PEComa) of the uterus: an outcome-based clinicopathologic analysis of 41 reported cases. Advances in Anatomic Pathology, 15(2), 63-75.

Pinto, A., Kahn, R. M., Rosenberg, A. E., et al. (2018). Uterine rhabdomyosarcoma in adults. Human Pathology, 74, 122-128.

Li, R. F., Gupta, M., Mc Cluggage, W. G., & Ronnett, B. M. (2013). Embryonal rhabdomyosarcoma (botryoid type) of the uterine corpus and cervix in adult women: report of a case series and review of the literature. The American Journal of Surgical Pathology, 37(3), 344-355.

Amant, F., Schurmans, K., Steenkiste, E., et al. (2004). Immunohistochemical determination of estrogen and progesterone receptor positivity in uterine adenosarcoma. Gynecologic Oncology, 93(3), 680-685.

Howitt, B. E., Sholl, L. M., Dal Cin, P., et al. (2015). Targeted genomic analysis of Müllerian adenosarcoma. The Journal of Pathology, 235(1), 37-49.

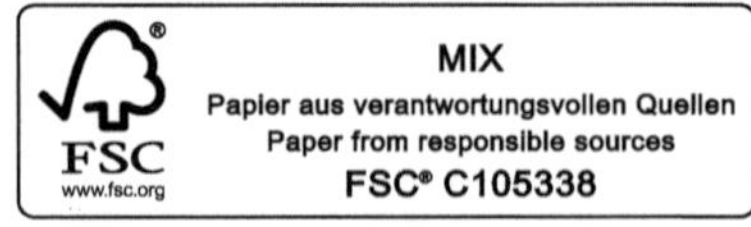

Printed by Books on Demand GmbH, Norderstedt / Germany